Master's Thesis

entitled

Understanding and Differentiating between Asperger's Syndrome and Autism Spectrum Disorder

By

Heather Wisen

Thesis Submitted in Partial Fulfillment of the Requirements for the Degree of Masters of Science in Healthcare Administration

Independence University

May 2019

Dedicated To:

Jeremy Coller, you have been an inspiration and I am proud of who you have become and what you have accomplished, and I am honored to be your mom.

Copyright © **2019**
Heather Wisen
This document is copyrighted material. Under copyright law, no parts of this document may be reproduced without the expressed permission of the author.

Approval Page

INDEPENDENCE UNIVERSITY

As members of the Final Project Committee, we certify that we have read the

document prepared

by

Heather Wisen

Understanding and Differentiating between Asperger's Syndrome and Autism Spectrum Disorder

and recommend that it be accepted as fulfilling the final project Requirement for the Degree of

Masters of Healthcare Administration

 Dr. Doret Ledford   Date: 05/07/2019
Dr. Doret Ledford, Course Instructor/AD/FPA

_____ Date:
05/09/2019
Dr. Carmen Herbel Spears RN DHA MSN BSN Dean of the School of Healthcare

Abstract

Asperger's since its original diagnosis has been classified many ways. It has ranged from its own disorder to being part of Autism and with new criteria it is being places as an Autism spectrum disorder and losing its own diagnosis as a syndrome. We looked at several studies that have been done that not only compare Asperger's to Autism but also to things such as high functioning autism, ADHD, and pervasive communication disorders. By comparing these studies, we can learn more about Asperger's and its relationship to these other disorders and determine the similarities. Studies used were surveys and questionaries' of parents who children were diagnosed with these disorders as well as an in-depth study of MRI images that show the brain development in each of these disorders and how they are different. From the studies utilized it is confirmed that while Asperger's and Autism do share similar traits they are indeed two entirely different disorders and should remain as so and not be classified under an umbrella term causing patients to miss out on treatment that could have assisted them better.

Keywords: Asperger's, Autism, ADHD, Communication Disorder, High-Functioning

Table of Contents

Abstract...vii

Table of Contents.......................................v

Chapter 1: Introduction..............................1
    Background of Study 1
    Problem Statement.............................7
    Purpose of the study..........................10
    Research Questions............................11
    Definition of Terms...........................13
    Summary...15

Chapter 2: Literature Review....................17
    Overview...17
    Summary...32

Chapter 3: Method....................................35
    Introduction....................................35
    Research Questions and Hypotheses...36
    Studies..38
    Study 1...38
    Study 2...47
    Study 3...50

Summary..................................51

Chapter 4: Results.............................53

    Purpose..................................53

    Descriptive Statistics....................57

    Study 1..................................57

    Study 2..................................62

    Study 3..................................66

    Summary Findings.......................75

Chapter 5: Discussion, Conclusion, Recommendations................................78

    Introduction..............................78

    Discussion................................82

    Recommendation for Action............87

    Recommendation for Future Study.....88

    Conclusion...............................90

References......................................92

List of Tables

Table 1: Neuro Behavioral Findings..................................……...…60

Table 2: Comparison between AD and ASD....67

List of Figures

Figure 1: Survey Questionnaire..................................40

Figure 2: Comparison of MRIs for Autism and Aspersers...65

Chapter 1: Introduction

Background of the Study

Asperger's Syndrome (AS) and Autism are considered milder than other levels of disability on the autism spectrum, but the most noticeable difference between the two is language (Angelsense, n.d.). Asperger's was first used as a diagnosis in 1940 by a Viennese Pediatrician names Hans Asperger. He observed children who had normal to above intelligence and language development yet also demonstrate autism like behaviors related to social and communication skills. Many professionals felt that Asperger's was a mild form of autism or a "High functioning: autism, however, in 1994 it became known as its own diagnosis.

Then again in 2013 it was reclassified in the DSM-5 under the umbrella term autism spectrum disorder (Autism Society, 2016). Asperger's was recently stripped away as a diagnosis and instead these individuals were classified as having an Autism Spectrum Disorder. Why was this change made and does Asperger's really fit into this new broad-spectrum category? Should it be labeled a social communication disorder as it has more of those properties then that of autism. To understand and answer these questions one must first understand the traits and characteristics of each, Asperger's, Autism, autism spectrum disorder and social communication disorders.

Autism covers a wide range of neurodevelopment disorders that are often characterized by things such as impairments with social behaviors and interactions, difficulty in verbal communication and body language, and patterns of repetitive behavior. Autism dates back into the 1880's and had been reclassified and more understood as studies have developed. It was officially added to the DSM-3 as the diagnosis criteria we know today. In 1991 schools began identifying students with this disorder and created a federal government category for special education. Social Communication disorder or SCD, is a newer addition to the DSM-5 as of 2013 and covers those individuals who suffer from problems related to social interactions, social understanding, and use of language in the proper context (Autism speaks, 2015). This diagnosis is based on both difficulties with verbal and nonverbal communication, such as, responding to others, taking turns when talking or playing, talking about emotions, staying on topic, adjusting speech to different situations, asking relevant questions and using proper word. SCD is similar to autism in that the both involve difficulty with social communication, however, Autism has more restricted and repetitive types of behaviors that go along side it.

Autism Spectrum Disorder, recently added as an umbrella term in the DSM-5 covers any individual who has difficulty with communication and interactions with others, Restricted interest and repetitive behaviors, and symptoms that interfere with one's ability to function in school, work, or other areas of life. With this umbrella term classifying all of the above disorders into one area, it would include anyone who displays symptoms such as:

- Making little or inconsistent eye contact or not looking at people when communicating
- Rarely sharing enjoyment of objects or activities

- Failing or being slow to respond to someone calling their name
- Having difficulties with back and forth conversation
- Often talking at length about a favorite subject without noticing that others are not interested
- Showing facial expressions or gestures that do not match what is being said
- Having a tone of voice that may sound sing-song, flat and robot-like when speaking
- Having trouble understanding another person's point of view on topics or being unable to predict or understand other actions

Other symptoms include repeating certain behaviors similar to and OCD manner or having unusual behaviors;

having a lasting intense interest in certain topics, overly focused interests; getting upset by changes in a routine;

Being more or less sensitive to sensory inputs, like light, noise, clothing textures, or temperatures

May experience sleep problems such as insomnia and suffer from irritability

Increase ability to learn things in detail and remember and retain information for extended periods of time or even years

Can be strong visual and auditory learners

Excelling in subjects such as math, science, music, or art (NIH, 2018)

Problem Statement

With Both similarities and differences, we must look at all aspects of Asperger's Syndrome and Autism and make a clear decision as to the proper way of differentiating between the two, as well as understanding why they should be classified individually and not as one umbrella diagnosis.

Background of the Problem

There have always been similarities between Asperger's and Autism, but they also have many differences. Comparing the two will help us better understand if they should be put into an umbrella term together. Children with autism are often uninterested in others while those with Asperger's want to interact with other but lack the know-how. They are social awkward and do not understand the rules of communication or do not understand things such as gestures and sarcasm. Autistic Children have interest in items such as a piece of string they always want to carry with them or that helps sooth them, while those that have Asperger's are interested or obsessed with topics and collecting, such as rocks, trains, and typewriters. They feel the need to be proficient in all the knowledge related to these topics to be subject masters. They may even be obsessed with things is history such as world war II and the titanic learning every aspect of these events.

One major difference between these two is speech. Most children diagnosed with autism have speech delays or are non-verbal. While those that have Asperger's have early verbal skills and tend to use large words. Speech patterns however may lack inflection or rhythm, may be formal but will be presented in a loud or high pithed tone, they may have issues understanding irony and humor and cannot engage in a give and take conversation (Autism Speaks, 2016). With so many areas and behaviors that now fit into this umbrella term, one must wonder if it is to generalize and those who have been given the diagnosis will be left without specialized care or services. Will anyone given the Autism Spectrum Disorder received the same generalized care as they are the generalized label? Looking at studies between the two groups we will be able to further understand the diagnosis process and the why these groups are being linked together. We will be able to answer questions about what services are available and what services will no longer be available with the new changes. The Studies that will be analyzed will also look at why a larger percentage of those previously diagnosed with asperser will no longer meet the criteria for the ASD and how this will affect those individuals.

Purpose of the Study

The Purpose of this study is to look at all aspects of Asperger's and Autism and analysis the differences that make them two different diagnosis. After review of secondary scholarly journals and articles we will be able to come to a conclusion as to the proper placement of each of these Disorders and determine if they are close enough in traits to be considered the same category of Autism Spectrum Disorder or to be known as they are currently as two separate diagnosis. With data collected from surveys as well as from MRI images the results will aide in the final determination that Asperger's should remain its own diagnosis with its own set of criteria.

Research Questions

Asperger's and Autism are two disorders are indeed different from one another

They are present both in the brain and in behavior traits differently and require different approaches from the medical field for treatment and diagnosis. The research questions asked are therefore:

1. Is Asperger's and Autism the truly the same thing?
2. Do these two disorders present in a similar manner and what areas if any do they share?

3. Should they be classified together as a spectrum disorder or be their own classification on the mental health Scale?

Research Hypothesis

The hypotheses that are created by these questions are as follows:

H1a: Asperger's and Autism are two disorders both present in the brain and are the same

H1o: Asperger's and Autism are two disorders both present in the brain and are the same

H2a: The medical treatment and diagnosis for Asperger's and Autism require different approaches.

H2o: The medical treatment and diagnosis for Asperger's and Autism require different approaches.

H3a: Asperger's individuals possess high more functioning IQ then those within the Autism spectrum

H3o: Asperger's individuals do not possess high and more functioning IQ then those within the Autism spectrum

Definitions of Terms

Asperger's - autism like behaviors related to social and communication skills

Autism- neurodevelopment disorder that are often characterized by things such as impairments with social behaviors, difficulty in verbal communication and patterns of repetitive behavior

DSM - Diagnosis and Statistical Manual of Mental Disorders, Number after refers to edition in which it appeared.

OCD - Obsessive Compulsive Disorder

Social Communication Disorder (SCD) - and covers a those who suffer from problems with social interactions, social understanding, and use of language in the proper context

Pervasive Developmental Disorders (PDD) - to a group of disorders characterized by delays in the development of socialization and communication skills

High-functioning autism (HFA) - is a term applied to people with autism who are deemed to be cognitively "higher functioning") than other people with autism.

Summary

Using all the information we have about the history of both Asperger's syndrome and Autism Spectrum Disorders, along with the information we have obtained from our research to help create the hypothesis, the questions needing answered can be closely looked at in the research that follows. The use of this information will aide in the final determination of where Asperger's and Autism differentiate from one another. We can see they have many similarities as well as difference's and can easily be mistaken as the same thing to the untrained person. With this information in which we have gathered we can easily explain, understand, and distinguish between the two disorders. Asperger's syndrome displays as a higher intelligence and broader use of vocabulary whereas Autism spectrum Disorders tend to result in lower IQ levels and, in most cases, non-verbal individuals. With this understanding we can differentiate the diagnoses.

Chapter 2: Literature Review

Overview

Asperger's Syndrome (AS) and Autism are considered milder than other levels of disability on the autism spectrum, but the most obvious difference between the two is language (Angelsense, n.d.). Asperger's has been a diagnosis since 1940 and just recently that was changed. The new diagnosis is Autism Spectrum Disorder. Is this truly a proper diagnosis? Are Asperger's and Autism the same thing and do they effect a person the same way. Several studies have been done that compare these two diagnoses and will help us to understand each and its relationships to one another if any, we will also look at the pathological research comparisons as well. An in depth look at these studies will help us to better understand and determine if

Asperger's truly is an Autism spectrum disorder. Studies showing changes in the brain both through autopsy and MRI imaging between the two groups could reveal a difference in the makeup of the brain. Studies of groups given various task will help set those with Asperger's aside from their counter parts who suffer from Autism Disorders.

Autism Diagnosis

Since there is much confusion as to the diagnosis of Autism Disorder and Asperger's Syndromes, several studies were done in an effort to examine the brain and investigate the differences between both. On study examined the brain of a 63-year-old Mathematician diagnosed with Asperger's show us that the how the development of the brain looks with one who was diagnosed with Asperger's. Clinical Summary shows a normal pregnancy and no contributing factors to autism or neurodevelopmental problems. It did show language and motor milestone met at an exceptional age. From Birth through adolescence he showed signs of repetitive behaviors, and strong interest and focus on one topic. As he grew up he would become angry when interfered with or given advise. He did not like changes in routine and would not travel because he would miss family lunch on Sunday. With his wide intellect he would read history and technical books and master the knowledge of the topic. He had an excellent memory and loved classical music. He began learning and master mathematics at a young age and by the age of 7 could do cubic roots, he had a strong grasp on algebraic expressions (Weidenheim, 2012).

The final study conducted on the brain upon his death suggested accelerated brain growth in the first few years of life then plateau to normal size in adulthood. When comparing this individuals' brain with images obtained through MRI they show comparable results. One study that was compared to what was observed was that of 18 high functioning Autism and 21 non-autistic males the study revealed MRI morphometry indicates that the enlarged brains of high functioning children with autism denote increased volume of the white matter. A possible explanation may be an increased number of narrower more tightly packed cortical microlumens found in the Asperger's group and was also associated with an increase of short interhemispheric connecting fibers and decrease of long input/output and interhemispheric myelinated axons (Weidenheim, 2012).

In 1940 when Asperger's was still a new diagnosis a study was done using children who demonstrated obsessive and repetitive behaviors, social deficits. Leo Kanner believed these children where similar to those who suffered schizophrenic behaviors (Sanders, 2009). However, during his study he found that those with Asperger's tended to be more obsessed with objects and avoided contact with people. Leo studied 11 children and, in the end, concluded the presents of autism and was used over the next thirty years as the base line of the autism diagnosis and even influenced the criteria used in the DSM-III. In the first two editions Autism was not considered to be a Mental Disorder. When they first appeared, they were referred to as Infantile Autism. Some still felt it was an early form of schizophrenic disorder. The original criteria for

Autism was Deficits in language, atypical patterns in speech lack of responsiveness to others, and unusable attachment to objects and unusual interest, a resistance to change. These criteria had to be met within the first 30 months of life to get the diagnosis. The next edition released added behaviors such as social interaction and communication impairments, and repetitive behaviors, interest, and activities, it also changed the diagnosis time frame to the age of 3. The only difference between a diagnosis of Asperger's and a diagnosis of Autism is there is no communication delay in those who have Asperger's.

Comparing Asperger Disorder and High Functioning Autism

There have been several studies done since 2000 that compare Asperger Disorder and High Functioning

Autism. With every new publication of the DSM the criteria changes and the differences between the two becomes smaller. Those that are diagnosed with the Asperger's Disorder tend to have an IQ of greater than 70. While those with High functioning Autism are lower. His study also suggest that those diagnosed with Asperger do well with verbal task, a study done by Ghaziuddin found that children diagnosed with autism were aloof and passive while those diagnosed with Asperger's were active but odd. The studies combine found that the diagnosing criteria for Asperger's regarding delays in speech are problematic because the delays are not specific nor well-defined, also a delay before age of three does not mean a lifelong impairment will be present, there comes in play that the language delay is left to the parent to decide, and this may not be accurately represented. With all the studies combined the language delay seems to be the discriminating variable between the diagnosis (Sanders, 2009).

The next study focused on the Difference of High functioning Autism and Asperger's Disorder based in Neuromotor behavior. Some believe the core diagnostic symptom for autism is neuromotor disfunction followed by social and communication impairments. A study was done with children who suffer from Autism and those diagnosed with Asperger's the study participants ranged in age from 7-18. The test subjects were given an assessment of intellectual function appropriate for their age based on the Wechsler Scale and then given nonverbal intellectual assessment based off the perceptual reasoning scale. The test subjects were measured on walking under the following criteria: speed per minute, steps per minute, stride length, distance from heel point to footfall. The findings of the study suggested involvement of the striatal and cerebellar motor circuits in autism (Nayate, 2012).

In contrast with autism, children with Asperger's Disorder displayed variable base of support that was present only during preferred walking (Nayate, 2012). Final findings of the study suggest that while autism and Asperger's Disorder are both associated with qualitatively distinct patterns of cerebellar and striatal disturbance as seen under conditions of low cognitive demand, when comparing the two in a more challenging conditions the low-level disturbances manifest as similar disorders of complex information processing. Clinically, these differences in low level neurobiology could possibly account for the behavioral distinction between the two disorders as well as the similarities in the complex cognitive functions such as their social interactions and repetitive behaviors (Nayate, 2012).

Researchers also examined different forms of test to look at similarities and differences between the groups. Comparison of scores from the Checklist for Autism spectrum, Childhood Autism Rating scale, Gilliam Asperger's Disorder scale for low and high functioning autism, Asperger's Disorder, ADHD, and typical development. Looking at all these scores we should be able to see a difference between each as well as any similarities they may have. The study consisted of 190 children with low functioning autism, 190 with high function autism or Asperger's, 79 with ADHD, and 64 typical children. The purpose of our study was to compare diagnostic agreement, reliability, and validity for three autism instruments that have some or most of these characteristics (Mayes, 2009). The first test was the Checklist for Autism Spectrum Disorder, the test based on a 20-minute interview with parents, teachers and caregivers. The questions asked are based on 30 symptoms of autism. In this study both those in the low functioning and high functioning groups scored in the autism range.

The Childhood Autism Rating scale was another vital test that help in helping to determine the diagnosis of Autism. The study that was done consisted of 15 items rated normal to severe. This test included physicians, special educators, and school psychologist. These raters based their responses on observations, parent reports, and relative medical records. Scores range from 16-60 with all scores 30 or higher to be considered autism range and are in agreeance with 87% of clinical diagnosis (Mayes, 2009). Gilliam Asperger's Disorder scale is a 32-item instrument and is completed by someone who has consistent contact with the subject. This Checklist is divided into 4 parts and then scored. If the subjects scores and 80 or above, they are considered to have Asperger's Disorder. The results of all the test came out that those with Low functioning autism scored 100 on checklist, 97 CARS, 88 GADS, High Functioning Scored 99 checklist 75 CARS, 92 GADS, and the ADHD group scored 0 checklist, 0 CARS, and 4 GADS, Typical scored 0 across the board. With this testing it is in agreement that criteria are valid for the testing.

Is High Functioning Autism Listed on the DSM?

Most people associate Asperger's with High function Autism, but this next study will compare the two and show differences between them. A study comparing Asperger to high functioning autism showed that High functioning autism is not listed in the DSM as an official diagnosis and falls under the general diagnosis of autism, but should it too have its own diagnosis? The study shows that Autism, ADHD, and Asperger's share a common genetic marker on chromosome 16 which has caused research to classify them together. Participants of this study were recruited from the autism society's registry and range in age from 5-17, there were 125 selected, theses test subject suffer either from Asperger's or High- functioning autism. The participants completed a 44-item survey that was broken down into 4 groups to measure interaction with others, speech, nonverbal communication and repetitive behaviors. Based on the study it was determined that out of the 125 that were part of this study 16 met the criteria for Asperger's, 15 met the criteria for high functioning autism and the remainder fell into the general autism category. The study finds differences between Asperger's and high functioning autism in that the Asperger's children had higher levels of psychopathology and were more anxious and had a high rate of anxiety disorders, were more likely to have Obsessive compulsive disorder, and depressive personalities (Thede, 2007).

Asperger's is no Longer Classified as an Autism Spectrum Disorder – People's Reaction

Recent studies how people react to the change that Asperger's is no longer classified as an autism spectrum disorder has shown that many families are leery of the diagnosis of autism spectrum disorder. This is mostly because autism has a negative perception, while Asperger's has a positive perspective and is linked to many geniuses such as Albert Einstein and Bill Gates. But the DSM changing the name and removing Asperger's those in which would have had the diagnosis and affiliation of such would rather fall under the negative autism perspective and therefore be looked down upon. The study of 547 showed that half of the participants were opposed to the change will 22% supported the change and 28% were uncertain (Kite,

2013). These 547 participants were asked various questions about autism and Asperger's and of the 547 a total of 491 felt there was a definitive difference between the two. 97% of social workers pathologist and nurses surveyed also indicated that they felt there was a difference between the two conditions. One fear that many involved in the study shared and was the second most asked question was would the change be beneficial in gaining services for clients who have Asperger's once they are classified under Autism spectrum disorder (Kite, 2013).

Summary

With all the available studies that have been done comparing these two Disorders it is evident that there is a large debate as to if they should carry the same classification. However, when looking at the scientific evidence as we did in the study of the brain and the MRI images we can see that there are differences in the brain for each of these disorders. It seems that both of these disorders are inherited and pasted through genetics yet do not present the same ways, even though both are present at birth. It can be seen that children diagnosed with Asperger's develop much faster at a younger rate as far as language skills and milestones while the autistic child lags behind and may never become verbal. For this reason alone, it should be said that Asperger's is its own diagnosis and not that of Autism. Just because Pervasive Disorders have some of the same common traits does not mean they should all be classified under the same umbrella term. You would not put Schizophrenia under autism so why classify Asperger's as such (Thede, 2007).

Further research and studies after the change is made in the DSM-5 will reveal more about the disorder and show the true spectrum of it at that time we will understand the differences more clearly. Asperger's will return as its own diagnosis because the intelligence level and IQ will not qualify it as Autism spectrum disorder.

Chapter 3: Methods

Introduction

Asperger's has been a diagnosis since 1940 and just recently that was changed. The new diagnosis as of 2013 is Autism Spectrum Disorder (Autism Society, 2016). Is this truly a proper diagnosis? Are Asperger's and Autism the same thing and do they effect a person the same way. Several studies have been done that compare these two diagnoses and will help us to understand each and its relationships to one another if any, we will also look at the pathological research comparisons as well. An in depth look at these studies will help us to better understand and determine if Asperger's truly is an Autism spectrum disorder. These studies come from secondary resources such as ProQuest scholarly articles.

This research will be utilizing pre-existing studies and mixed-methods in order to extrapolate qualitative information. The research questions asked are therefore:

4. Is Asperger's and Autism the truly the same thing?
5. Do these two disorders present in a similar manner and what areas if any do they share?
6. Should they be classified together as a spectrum disorder or be their own classification on the mental health Scale?

Research Hypothesis

The hypotheses that are created by these questions are as follows:

H1a: Asperger's and Autism are two disorders both present in the brain and are the same

H1o: Asperger's and Autism are two disorders both present in the brain and are the same

H2a: The medical treatment and diagnosis for Asperger's and Autism require different approaches.

H2o: The medical treatment and diagnosis for Asperger's and Autism require different approaches.

H3a: Asperger's individuals possess high more functioning IQ then those within the Autism spectrum

H3o: Asperger's individuals do not possess high and more functioning IQ then those within the Autism spectrum

Studies

Study One: Psychological and Neurobehavioral Comparisons of Children with Asperger's Disorder Versus High-Functioning Autism (2007)

Researchers investigated the personality and neurobehavioral differences between 16 children with diagnosis of Asperger's, 15 children who were classified as High functioning Autism or HFA, and 31 children as a control group. The ages of these participates ranged from 5 – 17 with mean age being 10. The study involved parents of these children as well as they rated their children's behaviors based on 44 items on an autistics symptoms survey as well a 200 item Coolidge Personality and Neuropsychological Inventory.

Participants were chosen from a registry obtained from the Autism Society of American. There were a total of 76 parents who offered to be part of the study which contained a 44-item survey of autistic symptoms and a 200 item Coolidge Personality and Neurobehavioral Inventory CPNI (Coolidge, 1998; Coolidge, Thede, Stewart, & Segal, 2002a).

The procedure used was the same the questionnaires that the parents of the all the children were asked to fill out and the results showed compared to the control group the Asperger's and HFA group had significantly elevated scores on the scale for the testing. It also showed There were more similarities than differences between the two groups when it came to the personality Scale although it did show with both scales that those with Asperger's scared very high in the areas for Anxiety compared to the HFA group and the control group (Thede, 2007). These will be investigated with more detail in the next chapter for further understanding.

Figure 1: Questionnaire

Survey of Autistic Symptoms

Please rate each item on the following scale. Try to answer how your child has behaved for most of his/her life or what appears to be characteristic of how your child acts most of the time.

1 = Strongly False

2 = More False Than True

3 = More True Than False

4 = Strongly True

Socialization

Speech & Language

1. My child has no close friends. _____

2. My child tends to avoid activities involving other children. _____

3. My child is a loner. _____

4. My child has trouble developing friendships with other children. _____

5. My child is socially clumsy or awkward. _____

6. My child has trouble understanding the feelings of others. _____

7. My child acts inappropriately with other children. _____

8. My child seems emotionally cold or detached. _____

9. My child approaches others only when he/she needs something for himself/herself. _____

10. My child points out things to me that he/she is interested in. _____

11. My child brings me things that he/she is interested in. _____

12. My child's speech development was delayed (e.g., not using single words by age 2 and unable to use simple phrases by age 3). _____

13. My child misinterprets what other people say. _____

14. My child has difficulty understanding common expressions such as "If looks could kill," "I'm history," or "Has the cat got your tongue?" _____

15. My child sounds like a "walking dictionary" or encyclopedia. _____

16. My child talks too much. _____

17. My child talks too little. _____

18. My child has trouble following conversations. _____

19. My child has a strange or unusual rhythm or inflection when he/she speaks_____

20. My child repeats over and over exactly what is said to him/her_____

21. My child misuses pronouns like substituting "I" for "you," "him" for "me," or "her" for "me." _____

22. My child has trouble starting or maintaining conversations with others. _____

23. My child has trouble playing like other children his or her age (for example, pretending or make-believe). _____

24. My child has limited use of gestures compared to other children. _____

25. My child has inappropriate or exaggerated facial expressions. _____

26. When talking to others, my child comes up too close to other people. _____

27. My child has a limited number of facial expressions compared to other children. _____

28. My child has large, clumsy or inappropriate body language or gestures. _____

29. My child is unable to give messages with his/her eyes. _____

30. My child has difficulty making or maintaining eye contact. _____

31. My child has a strange or weird handshake (or doesn't shake hands at all). _____

32. My child has trouble using his hands to express himself/herself. _____

33. My child has trouble reading other people's facial expressions. _____

34. My child is unaware of what he/she is communicating to others with his/her body language. _____

35. My child has trouble hugging or kissing people. _____

36. My child gets intensely interested or preoccupied with a single subject and doesn't seem to want to do anything else. _____

37. My child has to stick to some useless routine and gets angry if it is changed. _____

38. My child uses some hand or body gestures over and over (for example, hand flapping or finger twisting). _____

39. My child gets preoccupied or interested with parts of objects or just one aspect of a toy (for example, how it feels or a noise that it might make). _____

40. My child doesn't seem to be as interested in as many different things as other children. _____

41. My child is intensely fascinated with items involving transportation such as trains, planes, ships, cars, or roads. _____

42. My child has an intense dislike of change. _____

43. My child is exceptionally sensitive to lights, sounds, tastes, touch, or smells. _____

44. My child is uncoordinated or clumsy. _____

Study Two: Can Asperger syndrome be distinguished from autism? An anatomic likelihood meta-analysis of MRI studies (Date)

This Research was conducted by Kevin K. Yu, BSc; Charlton Cheung, PhD; Siew E. Chua, BM BCh; Gráinne M. McAlonan, MBBS, PhD and compares the MRI results of both those who have been diagnosed with Asperger's and those who have Autism. The study was conducted a systematic search for MRI studies of grey matter volume in people with autism. Studies with a majority of participants with an autism diagnoses and a history of language delay were assigned to the autism group. Those with an autism disorder but displayed no language delay were assigned to the Asperger syndrome group. The information obtained from the MRI Studies were then entered into anatomic likelihood estimation meta-analysis software with sampling size weighting to compare grey matter by Asperger syndrome or autism.

The procedure used to obtain these results was the comparison of multiple MRI images and then the results obtained were then entered into a special software which showed the following results which we will get into more detail on when we analyze this study further. The autism grey matter map showed lower volumes in the cerebellum, right uncus, dorsal hippocampus and middle temporal gyrus compared with controls; grey matter volumes were greater in the bilateral caudate, prefrontal lobe and ventral temporal lobe (YU, 2011). The Asperger syndrome indicated lower grey matter volumes in the bilateral amygdala/hippocampal gyrus and prefrontal lobe, left occipital gyrus, right cerebellum, putamen and precuneus compared with controls; grey matter volumes were greater in more limited regions, including the bilateral inferior parietal lobule and the left fusiform gyrus. Both Asperger syndrome and autism studies reported volume increase in clusters in the ventral temporal lobe of the left hemisphere (Yu, 2011).

Study Three: DSM-5 ASD Moves Forward into the Past (2014)

This research was done by Tsai in 2014. The study was an analysis of and comparative study on Asperger's and Autism. This study came about with the changes in the 5th edition of the DSM or Diagnostic and Statistical manual of Mental Disorders. The research consisted of 125 studies which compared the two. Of these 125 studies 30 concluded they were similar conditions while 95 of the studies found bot qualities and quantitative difference between the two. The research then furthered the exploration of this topic and compared 37 studies the compared Autism to Pervasive Developmental Disorder and found 9 that said there is no difference and 28 that again showed both qualitive and quantitative differences. Together these two research studies do not support the DSM 5th edition of grouping all the disorders into the category of Autism spectrum Disorder. Further analysis of this study will help us understand why these results are as they are and what lead the researcher to the final conclusions in which he reached.

Summary Analysis

All of the research has shown both similarities and difference between the Asperger sand Autism but is this research enough to say they are two different things? As we dig deeper into each of these studies will start to see the difference and be able to determine for ourselves if there is indeed a difference. This I a long going debate and much more research on both is going to come in the future as many feel the DSM 5th edition change is indeed a step backwards for the Autism and Asperger's community. Surveys and testing show significant difference as well as similarities the same outcome when comparing the MRI of the brain. Both of these Disorder mimic one another in traits yet the individuals who have been diagnosed are so different. There is not one-person with either of this Disorders that present the same as the other. Thing such as that are what makes this such a difficult disorder to understand and classify. With research we are going to try to make a distinction.

Chapter 4: Results

Purpose of the Study

Asperger syndrome is a developmental disorder characterized by significant difficulties in social interaction and nonverbal communication, it can also have repetitive patterns of behavior such as arm flapping or excitable jumping as well as very focused interests such as an interest in trains, cars or even vacuum cleaners. The diagnosis of Asperger's changed in 2013 when the diagnosis was removed from DSM-4 along with other previous mental health diagnosis and was be replaced by a single diagnostic category of autism spectrum disorders in DSM-5 (Brazian). In the DSM-5, the label of "Asperger's Syndrome" has been removed, however, the diagnosis itself remains only now with a new label, Social Communication Disorder, as a mild form of autism spectrum disorder (Autism Society, 2013). The DSM-5 text states "Individuals with a well-established DSM-IV diagnoses of autistic disorder, Asperger's disorder, or pervasive developmental disorder not otherwise specified should be given the diagnosis of autism spectrum disorder"(DSM-5).

Studies and research have been conducted by many individuals to determine the similarities and difference between Autism and Asperger's. With the most recent changes is the DMS 5th edition putting both disorders into one umbrella term has spark more interest in the topic of researching to find the difference and once again Bring Asperger's back as its own diagnosis. The studies we are going to look at will help to answer many questions that have been brought about on this topic and

55

help to understand the differences. The research questions asked are therefore:

7. Is Asperger's and Autism the truly the same thing?
8. Do these two disorders present in a similar manner and what areas if any do they share?
9. Should they be classified together as a spectrum disorder or be their own classification on the mental health Scale?

The hypotheses that are created by these questions are as follows:

H1a: Asperger's and Autism are two disorders both present in the brain and are the same

H1o: Asperger's and Autism are two disorders both present in the brain and are the same

H2a: The medical treatment and diagnosis for Asperger's and Autism require different approaches.

H2o: The medical treatment and diagnosis for Asperger's and Autism require different approaches.

H3a: Asperger's individuals possess high more functioning IQ then those within the Autism spectrum

H3o: Asperger's individuals do not possess high and more functioning IQ then those within the Autism spectrum

This chapter provides detailed data results of each of the studies utilized in this secondary study. With each set of written descriptive statistics illustrative or tables to help clarity of study findings. This chapter also concludes with a brief overview of the data presented in the Summaries.

Descriptive Statistics

Study One: Psychological and Neurobehavioral Comparisons of Children with Asperger's Disorder Versus High-Functioning Autism

This research consisted of an investigation of personality and neurobehavioral difference between 16 children with Asperger, 15 with High Functioning Autism, and 31 in a control group all ranging from 5-17 years of age (Thede, 2007). Asperger's is categorized as a pervasive developmental disorder and High Functioning Autism or HFA is a diagnosis that is used to describe and individual autistic disorder that have an IQ above the mentally retarded range and are verbally high functioning.

The 44-item survey of autistic symptoms was originally created to diagnose Autism, Asperger's, HFA, and pervasive developmental disorders per the criteria needed under the DSM. The items on this test cover areas such as socialization with others, this includes friend ships and social adaptiveness, it then ask about Speech with incudes delays, misinterpretations, inflection, and misuse pronouns, nonverbal communication is also questioned which includes gestures, facial expressions, and body language, Next there are questions that relate to receptiveness and stereotypical behaviors which can include things such as focused interest, repetitive gestures, intense dislike to change and sensitivity to stimuli, it also included questions about motor skills and clumsiness. Below is an example of the questions asked and the scale the parent is to use to rate each area.

The same parents where then given the 200-item inventory which is designed to assess Neurobehavioral deficits such as anxiety disorder, depression, oppositional defiant disorder and ADHD per the criteria in the DSM (Thede. 2007). Based the information obtained during this study it showed that 16 children met criteria for Asperger's Disorder meaning they showed no signs of language delay or mental retardation and had an IQ >70. 15 of the children met criteria for HFA meaning they had some language delays but not given the diagnosis of mental retardation. The table below breaks down the Neurobehavioral finding for each group based on the survey given:

Table 1: Neurobehavioral Findings

CPNI	Control	Asperger's	HFA
Generalized Anxiety Disorder	49.8	63.8	53.5
Oppositional Defiant Disorder	48.7	55.5	53.2
Major Depressive disorder	50	61.5	58.5
ADHD	50.2	69.6	66.1
Inattention	50.7	67	62.8
Hyperactivity / Impulsivity	47.3	67.8	65.9
Avoidance	49.9	60.8	50.6
Borderline	50.5	62.6	58.8
Conduct Disorder	50.7	48.3	50.0
Dependent	51.9	62.7	54.2
Depressive	47.7	56.1	44.2
Historic	49.6	57.5	55.5
Narcissistic	46	53.4	20.2
Obsessive Compulsive	47.9	65.5	53
Paranoid	49.3	49.8	43.6
Passive – aggressive	49.4	54.2	47.3

Schizotypal	51.8	72.5	78.4
Schizoid	51	68.4	71.9
Decision Making Difficulties	46	61.7	60.5
Metacognitive Problems	45.9	61.7	60.5
Social Inappropriateness	46.1	61.7	61.3

(Thede. 2007)

The final results of this study determined that the biggest difference between the Asperger's group and HFA was the increase in anxiety levels with Asperger's. It found no other evidence to determine that the two groups are distinguishably greater disruptiveness or motor clumsiness, it also went on to find the present study to support contentions that disorders in the autism spectrum may be associated with EF deficits such as the decision-making difficulties and ADHD. However, there was no evidence that the two clinical disorders may be distinguishable just on this basis.

Study Two: Can Asperger syndrome be distinguished from autism? An anatomic likelihood meta-analysis of MRI studies

This research was conducted to compare the gray matter of the brain seen on MRI report of those diagnosed with Asperger's and those diagnosed with Autism to see if there was a significant difference between the two groups. The method used to obtain this information for the study was through databases such as PubMed, the final results of all the paper reviewed where put into this study and give us the final conclusion. Once the information was gathered it was put into two groups those with Asperger's and those with autism based on language delays or no language delays. The autism group comprised of 9 studies and included 151 patients and 190 controls, the Asperger's group consisted of 9 studies and 149 patients with 214 controls. All diagnosis met the criteria placed in the DSM.

The autism studies generated a summary pattern of lower grey matter volumes in the cerebellum, right uncus, dorsal hippocampus and middle temporal, compared with controls; however, grey matter volumes were greater in numerous brain regions, including the bilateral caudate, prefrontal lobe and ventral temporal lobe (Yu, 2011).

The Asperger syndrome studies indicated that grey matter volumes were lower in the bilateral amygdala/ hippocampal gyrus regions, bilateral superior frontal gyri and left occipital gyrus compared with controls. Additional regions of lower grey matter volume were identified in the right hemisphere in the cerebellum, putamen, precuneus and medial frontal gyrus.

The meta-analysis of grey matter in people with Asperger's and autism revealed an overlap, as well as differences, between the two conditions. However, for both the Asperger and autism studies, it is noted the volume excess in the ventral temporal lobe of the left hemisphere around the middle and inferior temporal gyrus and lingual gyrus.

Below we can a see a comparison of these MRI's, The Autism scan is on the top and the Asperger's scan on the bottom.

Figure 2: Comparison of MRIs for Autism and Asperger's

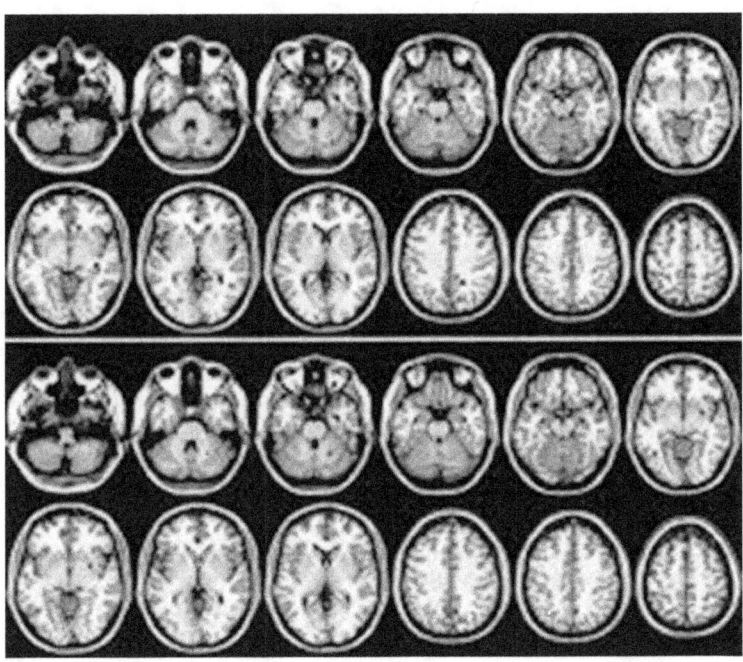

The conclusion of this study shows that there is gray matter differences between the two groups and that Asperger's sparser then those with autism and that Asperger's involves clusters of low gray matter volume in the left hemisphere while autism is more bilateral.

Both conditions hare clusters of gray matter in the left ventricle temporal lobe. These differences can be used in classifying these two groups differently as treatment would need to be altered depending on diagnosis.

Study Three: DSM-5 ASD Moves Forward into the Past

Research shows that autism has been part of the human condition since the mid-1300. (Tsai, 2014) This has been research and proven by several other researchers in history as we learned in previous chapters. This study used previous secondary studies to compare Asperger's, Autism, and Pervasive Developmental Disorders. These studies were accessed through PubMed, Medline, PsychInfo. Research articles for this study included those published in the Journal of Child Psychology and Psychiatry, Journal of Autism and

Developmental Disorders, and Research of Autism Spectrum Disorder (Tsai, 2014). Each research article was analyzed, and focus was placed on the comparison of these disorders.

A table showing the Comparison between AD and ASD can be seen on the next page, this chart from the study shows the outcome of analysis and what the final conclusion was based on the information.

Table 2: Comparison between AD and ASD

Author(s) (year)	Covered period	Number of studies reviewed	Variables studied	Conclusion
Myer and Minshew	1989 – 2000	14	IQ, cognition, language, motor skills, TOM, creativity, false	No difference between AD

(2002)			belief, recognizing mental state clinical characteristics, neuropsychological & language profiles, obstetric history and motor abnormalities, behavioral and psychiatric disturbance	and AsD
Howlin (2003)	1989-2001	26	IQ, cognition, language, motor skills, TOM, creativity, false belief, recognizing mental state clinical characteristics, neuropsychological & language profiles, obstetric history and	No difference between AD and ASD

			motor abnormalities, behavioral and psychiatric disturbance	
Macintosh and Dissanayake (2004)	1989-2003	41	IQ, cognitive profiles, language, echolalia, social cognition, social difficulty, global processing, TOM, visual-spatial skills, spatial cognition, motor function, movement preparation, diagnosis, comorbidities, obstetric history, genetic, epidemiology	No difference between AD and ASD
Sanders (2009)	2000 – 2008	16	IQ profiles, verbal ability, voice profiles, language	No difference betwee

				development, cognitive & symptom profiles, sensory-motor & cognitive functions self-presentational display rules, social interactions, social skills & problem behaviors, social phobia, diagnosis, follow-up and outcomes	n AD and ASD
Matson and Wilkins (2008)	1989 – 2007	22		Onset/develop mental, social interaction, communication, restricted or repetitive behaviors & interests, sensory-motor function, intellectual/ada ptive functioning,	ASD is a "distin ct disorder"

			psychopathology, general	
Kugler (1998)	1987 – 1996	18	Social skills, language, IQ profiles, cognition, diagnosis, motor function	ASD is a "distinct disorder"
Rinehart et al. (2002)	1996 – 2002	22	Neurocognitive, pedantic speech, neuropsychology, TOM, embedded figure test, the strange stories recognition of faux, belief, behavior & emotion, global processing, lateralization, visual illusion, shifting attention, neuropsych profiles movement, motor	Premature to exclude ASD from the DSM-5 ASD

			impairment, genetic, epidemiology, outcome	
Witwer and Lecavalier (2008)	1994 – 2006	22	IQ profiles, neuropsychological profiles, language measures, pedantic speech, sensory–motor & cognitive function, executive function, repetitive & stereotyped behavior and social disturbance, emotional/behavioral symptoms, depression and anxiety, anxiety & psychotic symptoms, psychiatric symptoms, early history,	Premature to exclude ASD from the DSM-5 ASD

			diagnosis, sex rates, follow-up and outcomes	
Kaland (2011)	1996 – 2010	11	Social behavior, pedantic speech, language development, IQ profiles, cognitive and symptom profile, cortical inhibition, cortical gyrification, diagnosis	Premature to exclude ASD from the DSM-5 ASD

(Tsai, 2014)

The DSM was developed for psychiatrists who were interested in describing and understanding the frequency with which mental illnesses developed in our society (Tsai, 2014). However, the DSM-II changed the approach and made it more of a criterion defining approach to enable doctors to make a diagnosis based on the symptoms of the patients. With all the research that has taken place surrounding the DSM it has also found very weak identifications and distinctions between mood disorders as well. The only risk seen with changes in the new DSM 5th edition is that eliminating the subtypes of PDD and ASD there will be an impact on the services and result in patients being denied services. A related issue in this study is diagnostic criteria for ASD, two things must remain constant and that is that rating scale cannot replace diagnostic criteria and that the gold standard remain that clinical diagnosis of autism remains just that, clinical.

This study found information leading to the DSM 5 changes stating that they were changed based on the findings in 2012 by Lord, who stated that "the best predictor of which autism spectrum diagnosis a person received was which clinic the individual went to, rather than any characteristic of the individual.". The ICD-11 has decided not to follow in the footsteps of the DSM and will continue to have subtypes such as Autism, Asperger's syndrome, Disintegrative disorder, and Rett syndrome and will not just use the classification of Autism Spectrum Disorder.

Summary of Findings

In conclusion of these studies our finding indicates that there is indeed a difference between Autism and Asperger's. We can see this difference in the study that compares the survey as it showed that there is indeed a difference in the mental health as well as motor skills and verbal skills between the two groups. Although some simulates are present it is apparent that they are not related. We see this again with the study that compares the MRI of the brain it shows changes in different areas. This alone should be enough evidence to differentiate the two as being their own disorder. If they truly were the same, then MRI images would indicate gray matter in the same places and they would have more similar traits then what they do. When looking at the final study of research on article of the change of umbrella terming them together we see there are conflicting studies showing them to be the same, very different, or not enough evidence to make the determination.

As medical professions one must step back look at the characteristic and from there determine if a patient fits the category of Autism or Asperger's and then off the proper treatment and services for that diagnosis. If they chose to treat all patients under the spectrum disorder category there will be losses of treatment and service that could have been otherwise provided to the individual.

Chapter 5: Discussion, Conclusion and Recommendations

Introduction

Asperger syndrome is a developmental disorder characterized by significant difficulties in social interaction and nonverbal communication, it can also have repetitive patterns of behavior such as arm flapping or excitable jumping as well as much focused interests such as an interest in trains, cars or even typewriters. The diagnosis of Asperger's changed in 2013 when the diagnosis was removed from DSM-4 along with other previous mental health diagnosis and was be replaced by a single diagnostic category of autism spectrum disorders in DSM-5. (Brazian,2018) In the DSM-5, the label of "Asperger's Syndrome" has been removed, however, the diagnosis itself remains only now with a new label, Social Communication Disorder, as a mild form of autism spectrum disorder. (Autism Society, 2016) The DSM-5 text states "Individuals with a well-established DSM-IV diagnoses of autistic disorder, Asperger's disorder, or pervasive developmental disorder not otherwise specified should be given the diagnosis of autism spectrum disorder" (DSM-5). A study, published in April 2012 using a preliminary version of the new DSM-5 autism spectrum criteria found about 75 percent of patients who had been diagnosed with Asperger's under the old criteria would no longer qualify for a diagnosis, raising the possibility that they could lose access to services, such as special education in schools. However, those diagnosed before the change in 2013 will get to keep their diagnosis (Luts, 2018).

Three studies were utilized to determine the differences between Asperger's and Autism. The research questions asked are therefore:

10. Is Asperger's and Autism the truly the same thing?
11. Do these two disorders present in a similar manner and what areas if any do they share?
12. Should they be classified together as a spectrum disorder or be their own classification on the mental health Scale?

The hypotheses that are created by these questions are as follows:

H1a: Asperger's and Autism are two disorders both present in the brain and are the same

H1o: Asperger's and Autism are two disorders both present in the brain and are the same

H2a: The medical treatment and diagnosis for Asperger's and Autism require different approaches.

H2o: The medical treatment and diagnosis for Asperger's and Autism require different approaches.

H3a: Asperger's individuals possess high more functioning IQ then those within the Autism spectrum

H3o: Asperger's individuals do not possess high and more functioning IQ then those within the Autism spectrum

Discussion

My personal connection to this topic was due to my son being diagnosed at the early age of 3 with Asperger's, these individuals are fascinating to learn from. Having worked with several areas of special needs there is so much we have yet to learn about each area of Autism. By not classifying them all as Autism Spectrum and just leaving each as its own diagnosis and would allow many more doors to open for these individuals, many people see autism and automatically think of it as a non-verbal low intelligence while these individuals who suffer Asperger's are normally above average intelligence. We saw this with the study that was discussed in the previous chapters.

Asperger's from what I have witnessed over the last 14 years is an amazing gift. It should not be referend to as a disorder as it is far from fitting that description. The only challenges these individuals face on a daily basis is the ability to fit in. They lack some social skills, which we saw was referred to as pervasive communication disorder. The individuals are just attracted so to speak to one topic and do not understand laws of communication. Most are a book of knowledge and should be given the privilege to be known for what they are and not be umbrellaed into a category with such a broad spectrum.

    In this research we learned what advantages and disadvantages there are for the change in diagnosis. Aspies as they refer to themselves as are highly intelligent individuals and some even considered gifted. This topic applies to real life as these are people who walk about with us and are achieving amazing thing.

Several scientists, physicist, actors, and many others have suffered this disease and made huge impacts in our society. The shared diagnosis gave the kids who had it someone to look up to, to strive to be just as great knowing they could accomplish great things despite a diagnosis.

Interpretation of the Findings

The materials used for this Thesis were secondary studies that have been done on the topic. The materials in the studies mostly consisted of surveys and questionnaires which include but are not limited to: IQ testing, Neuromotor skills testing, assessment of intellectual function appropriate for their age based on the Wechsler Scale and then given nonverbal intellectual assessment based off the perceptual reasoning scale, Checklist for Autism Spectrum Disorder, Childhood

Autism Rating scale, and the Gilliam Asperger's Disorder scale just to name a few. After looking at all the studies done on each of these individuals from Asperger's, Autism, and high functioning Autism we can definitely conclude that watch of them is interesting in their own ways. The studies we looked at showed that while they do have some similarities they have several differences as well.

The study that showed the greatest difference between these disorders was study two in chapter 4. As we can see from analyzing the results of what disorders stem from each of these we can see that Asperger's has a higher rate of issues such as Anxiety, Depression, ADHD, Narcissistic, Obsessive compulsive, Passive aggressive, Schizotypal, schizoid, Decision making, and social impartments (Thede. 2007). With Such distinct differences how can one say they should be placed under the umbrella term of Autism Spectrum? Based on these finding they should remain their own diagnosis and care plan being specialized for their care as that for Autism would not benefit these individuals as we saw in an another study most people who are diagnosed Asperger's Syndrome have and IQ about 70 while those with Autism are diagnosed with and IQ below 60. How would the same treatment work for both groups if placed under this generalized term (Thede, 2007).

Another study that showed a difference between these two syndromes or disorder is the results that was found from the analysis of the MRI. It showed us that there are distinct differences between the brain make up of each of these disorders and that those with Asperger's have a faster development in the brain at an early age leading to the early ability to speak and the use of larger words. As it showed us that changed in gray matter are in different places in the brain which effects the outcome of thought, speech, and intelligence (Yu, 2011). The Aspies had gray matter volumes were lower in the bilateral amygdala/ hippocampal gyrus regions, bilateral superior frontal gyri and left occipital gyrus which was more sparse then those with Autism (Yu, 2011).

Recommendation for Action

Recommendation for how we can address this issue currently would be to leave things are they were before the change in 2013 to the DSM-5 that took the Asperger's Syndrome diagnosis away. By having this diagnosis doctors and specialist were able to offer more resources to those who had been given the Asperger Syndrome Diagnosis. If brought back these individuals would continue to stand out as their own disorder and not be classified as Autism Spectrum Disorders and therefore miss out on the available resources for Asperger's. With the umbrella classification they are currently falling under resources are either limited or absent all together as most of the previous patients given the Diagnosis of Asperger's no longer meet the new criteria as discussed earlier in this research and are not given the treatment they are needed. The diagnosis must come back so these individuals can receive proper treatment and resources they need to live productive lives and grow as an individual.

Recommendation for Future Research

The studies examined showed that further research should be conducted but until those studies are done the DSM 5 should not changes. There are too many controversial issues relate to this topic being so new and they need to be analyzed and studied further. If any changes should ne made it should be to make Asperger's, its own entity with in this so widely used publication for diagnosis criteria. As far as future research is concerned the recommendation would be a closer observation group over a wider time frames as opposed to just written questionnaires. But observing quality of life and observer can see differences and recommend better treatment and criteria for diagnosis. To understand those that so called suffer from Asperger's, Autism or High functioning Autism one must really analyze every part of their daily living. It would be an amazing research project to spend a few years learning the traits instead of going by past writings based of doctor's diagnosis out of a criteria book that is changed on how society wants to view the syndrome at that time.

Conclusion

Asperger's are amazing individuals as are those who suffer and disorder by in summary they deserve to be seem for who they truly are, amazing individuals within our society. Even those these individuals share common ground with other disorders they are breed within their own. To get to come across someone who has grown up with this syndrome the average person would be amazed by their genius personalities and knowledge. So instead of grouping everyone who is deferent into an umbrella term we as a society need to learn and embrace each of them as the individual they are. Just because one person has Asperger's or Autism does not mean everyone you meet who has that diagnosis is the exact same. As results showed everyone is different and deserves to be see and acknowledged as so.

References

Adams, M. P. (2013). Explaining the theory of mind deficit in autism spectrum disorder. Philosophical Studies, 163(1), 233-249.doi:http://dx.doi.org/10.1007/s11098-011-9809-z

Autism Society, (2016) Asperger's Syndrome, Retrieved from: http://www.autism-society.org/what-is/aspergers-syndrome/

Badone, E., Nicholas, D., Roberts, W., & Kien, P. (2016). Asperger's syndrome, subjectivity and the senses. *Culture, Medicine and Psychiatry.* 40(3), 475-506.

doi:http://dx.doi.org/10.1007/s11013-016-9484-9

Barahona-Corrêa, J. B., & Filipe, C. N. (2016). A concise history of aspergers syndrome: The short reign of a troublesome diagnosis. Frontiers in Psychology. (6), 2024. doi:10.3389/fpsyg.2015.02024

Bazian, (December 4, 2012), Asperger's not in DSM-5 mental health manual, NHS, retrieved from: https://www.nhs.uk/news/mental-health/aspergers-not-in-dsm-5-mental-health-manual/

Fine, L., & Myers, J. W. (2004). Understanding students with asperger's syndrome. *Phi Delta Kappa Fastback.,* (520), 3-39. Retrieved from https://search.proquest.com/docview/203654515?accountid=41759

Kite, D. M., Gullifer, J., & Tyson, G. A. (2013). Views on the diagnostic labels of autism and asperser's disorder and the proposed changes in the DSM. *Journal of Autism and Developmental Disorders.* 43(7), 1692-700. doi:http://dx.doi.org/10.1007/s10803-012-1718-2

Kulage, K. M., Smaldone, A. M., & Cohn, E. G. (2014). How will DSM-5 affect autism diagnosis? A systematic literature review and meta-analysis. *Journal of Autism and Developmental Disorders.* 44(8), 1918-32. doi:http://dx.doi.org/10.1007/s10803-014-2065-2

Lai, W. W., Goh, T. J., Oei, T. P., S., & Sung, M. (2015). Coping and well-being in parents of children with autism spectrum disorders (ASD). *Journal of Autism and Developmental Disorders.* 45(8), 2582-2593. doi:http://dx.doi.org/10.1007/s10803-015-2430-9

Lauritsen, M. B. (2013). Autism spectrum disorders. *European Child & Adolescent Psychiatry.* 22, 37-42. doi:http://dx.doi.org/10.1007/s00787-012-0359-5

Lehti, V., Cheslack-postava, K., Gissler, M., Hinkka-yli-salomäki, S., Brown, A. S., & Sourander, A. (2015). Parental migration and asperger's syndrome. *European Child & Adolescent Psychiatry.* 24(8), 941-948. doi:http://dx.doi.org/10.1007/s00787-014-0643-7

Mayes, S. D., Calhoun, S. L., Murray, M. J., Morrow, J. D., Yurich, K. K., L., . . . Petersen, C. (2009). Comparison of scores on the checklist for autism spectrum disorder, childhood autism rating scale, and Gilliam asperger's disorder scale for children with low functioning autism, high functioning autism, asperger's disorder, ADHD, and typical development. *Journal of Autism and Developmental Disorders.* 39(12), 1682-93. doi:http://dx.doi.org/10.1007/s10803-009-0812-6

Mazefsky, C. A., & Oswald, D. P. (2007). Emotion perception in asperger's syndrome and high-functioning autism: The importance of diagnostic criteria and cue intensity. *Journal of Autism and Developmental Disorders.* 37(6), 1086-95. doi:http://dx.doi.org/10.1007/s10803-006-0251-6

Montgomery, C. B., Allison, C., Lai, M., Cassidy, S., Langdon, P. E., & Baron-Cohen, S. (2016). Do adults with high functioning autism or aspersers syndrome differ in empathy and emotion recognition? *Journal of Autism and Developmental Disorders.* 46(6), 1931-1940.

doi:http://dx.doi.org/10.1007/s10803-016-2698-4

Nayate, A., Tonge, B. J., Bradshaw, J. L., Mcginley, J. L., Iansek, R., & Rinehart, N. J. (2012). Differentiation of high-functioning autism and Asperger's disorder based on neuromotor behaviour. *Journal of Autism and Developmental Disorders.* 42(5), 707-17.

doi:http://dx.doi.org/10.1007/s10803-011-1299-5

Ohan, J. L., Ellefson, S. E., & Corrigan, P. W. (2015). Brief report: The impact of changing from DSM-IV 'asperger's' to DSM-5 'autistic spectrum disorder' diagnostic labels on stigma and treatment attitudes. Journal of Autism and Developmental Disorders, 45(10), 3384-3389. doi:http://dx.doi.org/10.1007/s10803-015-2485-7

Peterson, C. C., PhD., Garnett, M., Kelly, A., & Attwood, T. (2009). Everyday social and conversation applications of theory-of-mind understanding by children with autism-spectrum disorders or typical development. European Child & Adolescent Psychiatry, 18(2), 105-15. doi:http://dx.doi.org/10.1007/s00787-008-0711-y

Rinehart, N. J., Tonge, B. J., Bradshaw, J. L., Iansek, R., Enticott, P. G., & McGinley, J. (2006). Gait function in high-functioning autism and asperger's disorder. *European Child & Adolescent Psychiatry.* 15(5), 256-264. doi:http://dx.doi.org/10.1007/s00787-006-0530-y

Rudy, L. J. (November 22, 2018), Does Asperger's still Exist? Very well health, Retrieved from https://www.verywellhealth.com/does-asperger-syndrome-still-exist-259944

Ruiz Calzada, L., Pistrang, N., Mandy, W. P., & L. (2012). High-functioning autism and asperger's disorder: Utility and meaning for families. Journal of Autism and Developmental Disorders, 42(2), 230-43. doi:http://dx.doi.org/10.1007/s10803-011-1238-5

Samson, A. C., Huber, O., & Ruch, W. (2011). Teasing, ridiculing and the relation to the fear of being laughed at in individuals with asperger's syndrome. Journal of Autism and Developmental Disorders, 41(4), 475-83. doi:http://dx.doi.org/10.1007/s10803-010-1071-2

Sanders, J. L. (2009). Qualitative or quantitative differences between Asperger's disorder and autism? historical considerations. Journal of Autism and Developmental Disorders, 39(11), 1560-7. doi:http://dx.doi.org/10.1007/s10803-009-0798-0

Spikins, P. (2009). Autism, the integrations of 'difference' and the origins of modern human behaviour. *Cambridge Archaeological Journal.* 19(2), 179-201.

doi:http://dx.doi.org/10.1017/S0959774309000262

Simpson, R. L., & Brenda, S. M. (1998). Aggression among children and youth who have asperger's syndrome: A different population requiring different strategies. *Preventing School Failure.* 42(4), 149. Retrieved from https://search.proquest.com/docview/228443531?accountid=41759

Thede, L. L., & Coolidge, F. L. (2007). Psychological and neurobehavioral comparisons of children with asperger's disorder versus high-functioning autism. *Journal of Autism and Developmental Disorders.* 37(5), 847-54. doi:http://dx.doi.org/10.1007/s10803-006-0212-

Van Steensel, F. J., A., Bögels, S., M., & de Bruin, E. I. (2015). DSM-IV versus DSM-5 autism spectrum disorder and social anxiety disorder in childhood: Similarities and differences. *Journal of Child and Family Studies.* 24(9), 2752-2756. doi:http://dx.doi.org/10.1007/s10826-014-0078-2

Weidenheim, K. M., Escobar, A., & Rapin, I. (2012). Brief report: Life history and neuropathology of a gifted man with aspergers syndrome. *Journal of Autism and Developmental Disorders.* 42(3), 460-7. doi:http://dx.doi.org/10.1007/s10803-011-1259-0

Young, R. L., & Rodi, M. L. (2014). Redefining autism spectrum disorder using DSM-5: The implications of the proposed DSM-5 criteria for autism spectrum disorders. *Journal of Autism and Developmental Disorders*, 44(4), 758-65.

doi:http://dx.doi.org/10.1007/s10803-013-1927-3

www.ingramcontent.com/pod-product-compliance
Lightning Source LLC
Chambersburg PA
CBHW072155170526
45158CB00004BA/1655